In a New York Minute

IN A NEW YORK MINUTE...

Everything Did Change

PAULA F. GUINNIP,

MD, FACS, FCCP, OSF

ISBN: 9798674871187

Prologue

This book isn't meant to be a technical medical guide on the management of the beta coronavirus SARS-CoV-2 or its resulting disease, COVID-19 (coronavirus disease 2019). The purpose of this book is to share my experiences treating patients in one of the most affected areas of the United States—New York City. It is also a story of what I was feeling as this played out. After watching the devastation on the news and hearing the voices of despair, I could no longer watch tacitly at a distance: I felt compelled to volunteer my services. I hope that my story can shed light on some of the unusual characteristics of this illness and further help others on the front lines.

This book is about heroism of a cardiac surgeon, who adapted her training and became an intensivist, volunteering to work in a major institution in New York City that was treating Covid-19 patients This at a time when little was known about this pandemic. She left behind her family, at tremendous personal risk, to offer her services to help the people of New York, which was described as the epi-center of Covid-19 pandemic. The book describes the pain and suffering, not only by patients and their families, but also by first responders, nurses and physicians who were treating these critically ill patients. In scenes vividly described, this book gives the reader a feeling of the agony of those who were risking their lives to help unfortunate Covid-19 patients, some at brink of death, with no specific treatment available. Not only the people from New York, but also the public in general, will feel the impact that this pandemic had on the personal lives of patients, their families, first responders, nurses physicians and all allied personnel. This book will document for the future generation the resilience and strength of the people of New York and those who answered the call the action to treat Covid-19 patients.

—Professor Tomas Antonio Salerno, MD

1

1966. It is autumn in Syracuse, New York, when Bob and Phyllis Flummerfelt welcome to the world their brand-new baby, Paula Michele, on Tuesday, October 18. Both sets of grandparents are present from the start at the birth in St. Joseph's Hospital in Syracuse, and the newlyweds officially become a family.

Hello. This is Paula. This is my story of coming into the world and growing up in upstate New York. Looking at what is going on in my life right now, it all makes sense: I ended up just where I was supposed to. My parents raised me in Auburn, New York, and my grandparents—Elizabeth and Sam and Ruth and Beecher—played a pivotal role in my upbringing. A few key events got the ball rolling for my medical career.

Studious and inquisitive, I essentially began my medical journey in the summer before fourth grade at Seymour Library. I remember wanting to go to the library over going any other place. I considered athletics a complete waste of time and spent all my time playing the piano and reading medical books. I was only interested in studying to become a doctor. I am not sure why. No one in the family had gone to medical school, but my family supported me one hundred percent once they knew how much it meant to me.

I was annoyed when I was required to learn how to swim. *What a waste of time this is going to be!* I had put off learning how to swim so long that I had to start in the YMCA's polliwog class with first graders. By then I was nine! I was so embarrassed, and it was very important to me to act as though I had been swimming for a long time. I continued my classes until I achieved the highest status of "porpoise." I remember my instructor to this day. Randy, who probably felt sorry for me, was as gentle on me as possible. He was the only swim teacher there, so he accompanied me on my journey right from the beginning.

When I was not in the pool, however, I was reading. My mother thought I should be reading *Johnny Tremain* at my age, but I had no interest in doing so and instead feasted my eyes on *Grey's Anatomy*. I read the book cover to cover that summer. Yes: that was all I wanted to do. My mother kept harping on my book choices, though.

My mother was a consummate educator and a sixth-grade math teacher, so I felt I had to perform at a higher level in school than the other kids. I did not want to embarrass her. So I made library trips a summer ritual and even started working there as a page when I was fourteen. I was not only reading medical books but also getting ahead with the next year's curriculum.

Our planned family trips for summer vacations got to be a drag. I remember enduring a trip to Lake Placid and the North Pole. My parents tried to get me excited about seeing Santa Claus and the future site of the 1980 Winter Olympics, and I just wanted to study. As I got older, it just got worse. During a trip to the United Kingdom, I don't think I even got out of the car! For some odd reason I felt like I always had to study, and I still feel the same way today. I just want to learn more and pass it on to others. But back then I was under a lot of pressure to succeed—pressure I placed on myself.

2

My fellow classmates at Owasco Elementary School in Cayuga County, upstate New York, were a talented group of overachievers as well. We did the usual kid events like going to each other's birthday parties, but we were intensely competitive with one another. We were Ivy-League-bound! Cornell University was only thirty-eight miles from my home on First Avenue in the town of Owasco, and that was where I was going! Of the top ten students in my high school class, four of us went to Cornell, and the others went to Harvard University, Massachusetts Institute of Technology, and Rensselaer Polytechnic Institute. The competition was huge!

I gained my undergraduate degree in biology at Cornell University in Ithaca, New York. I never wanted to leave after the four years. How wonderful is it to have the guy who wrote the organic chemistry or biology textbook as your professor? How great is it to have Nobel laureates as your teachers? But the downside was that just about everyone I interacted with had been valedictorian of their high school class, so the competition grew fiercer. The margin to succeed was slim.

I hate to admit that I was not accepted to Weill Cornell Medical College. I was devastated. I have nothing against State University of New York (SUNY)–Binghamton, but my mother would try to comfort me by saying that had I gone there, I would have obtained a higher GPA and gotten into Cornell for med school. With gratitude, I was accepted to Georgetown University School of Medicine in 1988. I took great comfort in the fact that it was a Jesuit school, and everyone knows Jesuits are the academicians, right? I loved the academics at Georgetown, and many of the instructors and professors were from the National Institutes of Health (NIH) and the Armed Forces Institute of Pathology. Plus, the diversity of the metropolitan DC area made the learning environment robust.

Georgetown turned out to be the right place for me, but it was not New York. I had never left the state before, and it was hard to deal with the travel distance from home and with being away from my family for the first time.

When I matched to a residency program in anatomic and clinical pathology at the University of Rochester in New York, I quickly realized I wasn't at Georgetown anymore. It had not dawned on me until then that my career choice would rarely allow me to see any patients. My avid love for learning had caused me to gravitate to pathology, but my love for doing things with my hands was leading me to be a surgeon. I withdrew from the pathology residency, reapplied to general surgery, and had to undergo the match program all over again. The others around me didn't know how to respond. It was a risk, certainly, but I knew it was a risk I had to take. And it was fine! I never doubted I would get a spot in general surgery.

I interviewed widely on the East Coast, from Massachusetts to Pennsylvania, and I matched at SUNY–Buffalo. I would rather have continued at Rochester, but I decided this would be my home for the next seven years.

It was not customary for my family to venture west of Auburn. Truthfully, the only reason I even interviewed at Buffalo was because my parents had brought me along for the fun of it to attend the first Bills game in Buffalo's new stadium (Bills versus the Washington Redskins). Buffalo was new territory for me.

Surgical residency in Buffalo was quite the challenge back in the 1990s. A lot of world experts were attending, and the standards were sky-high. Every resident feared Dr. Frank Booth, a critical care surgeon, as if he might crush us. We really had to "know our stuff." Looking back, I realize how much he taught me about ventilators, hyperalimentation, tracheostomies, and treating deadly infections. At that time, as we tried to treat several bad cases of AIDS, we were listening to guidelines from Dr. Anthony Fauci and reading constantly.

Buffalo was a special place for me because that is where I was introduced to my mentor, Dr. Tomas Salerno. He arrived in Buffalo in 1994 from Toronto. A revolutionary heart surgeon, he was teaching the heart surgeons at Buffalo General Medical Center new ways of doing surgery—with the heart moving. The gold standard up to that time had been to arrest the heart (keep it still with cardioplegia) before sewing on grafts. Dr. Salerno's method was called "warm heart surgery," and he wrote the book. If not for him, I would not be writing this book today, nor would I have become one of a very select group of woman heart surgeons. (The first woman heart surgeon was Dr. Nina Braunwauld, also from New York, and she was one of my role models. For me, Dr. Salerno was the male version of her.)

I had met Dr. Salerno during my general surgery rotation on cardiac service, and I worked with him as much as I could.

At the end of that rotation, in what would become a pivotal moment of my career, he asked me, "Would you ever want to be a heart surgeon? I think you have what it takes."

I had never thought I could achieve all that he had achieved, but true to his promise, he accepted me into the second-most competitive cardiac program in New York state in 1996, and I started July 1, 1998. My grandmother gave me white roses that day to celebrate my achievement.

So when he encouraged me to write this book about how it was for me to drop what I was doing and return to New York to help fight COVID-19, how could I say no?

3

In March of 2020, I was trying to build a new thoracic surgical practice in Missouri as an employed physician and had just started a full-time surgical job a few weeks prior. I was working in Missouri, away from home in Oklahoma, but I had not permanently moved there yet.

For the past year, I had been planning to go on spring break to Walt Disney World in Orlando with my son's marching band. I drove home to Tahlequah, Oklahoma, and on March 10 all 150 of us packed onto the buses. I had a pit in my stomach, though, and sensed that this trip would not happen.

On March 11 the World Health Organization (WHO) declared COVID-19 a pandemic; the National Basketball Association suspended its season; Oklahoma State University, the University of Oklahoma, and Northeastern State University had all just canceled their semesters; and our bus to Orlando turned around and brought us home. By the end of March, our country was on lockdown.

Lockdown? That won't be for me, an essential worker, I thought. I expected I would have to start working as a staff member in the coronavirus units in my Oklahoma hometown and in the town of my then-current practice in Missouri. But no one called me in to work. *But people are dying, and they need doctors, right?* Instead of receiving an emergent phone call asking me to come help, I got notified that all surgery was being shut down and that I didn't have a job. That hit me hard. I understood why surgery was not safe, but surely I would still be needed, I had thought.

With no work, I became very depressed. I started watching the television, and soon New York Governor Andrew Cuomo's cry for help caught my attention. One particular afternoon I remember intently watching Governor Cuomo on the television. He was literally begging doctors to come to New York to help treat the many patients afflicted with COVID-19. He looked scared.

I felt horrible. *Here I am, sitting on the couch, doing nothing. The place I work does not want me, and my local hospital does not need me.* At that time, the number of cases was extremely low in Missouri and Oklahoma in comparison to New York City. *But my old stomping ground needs my help.*

On that very day—March 27, 2020—I received an email addressed to all licensed New York state physicians from Governor Cuomo:

March 20, 2020

Dear Health Professional:

We need the help of additional qualified health professionals and related professionals to supplement our hospital capacity on a temporary basis to treat seriously ill coronavirus patients including those that may need to be intubated.

If you are available, we need the following information immediately:

- Your specific qualifications and experience

- Date of last certification and license

- Last date of practice

- Role in last practice

- Contact information including location

- Current age

- Would you be willing to work in other parts of New York State?

- Describe your interest and ability to be able to provide your services to treat patients if the need should arise in the future.

Paula Michele Guinnip, MD, FACS, FCCP, OSF

....

Please provide these responses within 36 hours using this survey: https://www.health.ny.gov/assistance. If you have any questions please contact workforce@exec.ny.gov. Your immediate attention is necessary and appreciated.

With your help, New York State is working to protect our residents and strengthen our public health system to deal. We appreciate your commitment to the health and safety of all New Yorkers and look forward to building on our partnership.

Michael Dowling, President & CEO of Northwell Health, and Kenneth Raske, President, Greater New York Hospital Association, are leading this "surge project" for me and I hope you cooperate. It is as important an issue as we have ever seen.

Sincerely,

ANDREW M. CUOMO

Yes, I was still licensed. I had kept my New York license active for twenty-six years despite not working there for twenty. I didn't know why, but perhaps this was the reason.

So I made a quick inventory of the requirements: Could I go to what was becoming the US epicenter of the pandemic? Would I be helpful? Did I have enough critical care experience? *Of course! I'm a cardiothoracic surgeon!* Did I know how to intubate patients, and could I do it safely over and over again? Would I know how to treat their pathology? In a split second, I realized I was qualified, and immediately I responded and volunteered my services.

I had a choice to go anywhere in New York City, and I wanted to go where I felt would be the hardest hit—the Bronx. Since 2017, while working with many pulmonary-critical-care specialists, I had obtained significant ventilator-unit experience and had learned skills needed to take care of COVID-19 patients. Plus, this was a brand-new virus, and no one was an expert. I felt that my three years in a long-term acute-care hospital in Missouri were a good foundation.

So I threw my hat in the ring! I waited for a response, and on April 18 I got the phone call.

4

ON APRIL 16, 2020, I received the phone call at 2:12 p.m. (CDT) in Tahlequah, Oklahoma. The caller ID said "New York, New York." *This might be the hospital calling.* My mouth went dry.

"Hi, this is Paula Guinnip."

"I'm Dr. Chinyere Anyaogu from North Central Bronx Hospital. Please just call me Chi-Chi," said the woman on the other end. "I am calling to see if you are still willing to come to New York City."

Before I could answer, she went on, saying that things had really gotten worse and that many of the patients with COVID-19 had renal failure. "Our units are exploding, but we have new makeshift units to put the patients who are overflowing. What we really need right now are trained physicians." She continued, "You indicated on the volunteer form that you wanted to come here and volunteer. Do you still want to come volunteer?"

"Yes, ma'am, I do." I asked her when she needed me to be there.

"Right now," she said. She instructed me to book the first flight I could find; reservations would be complimentary. Later this afternoon, the coordinating group would send me a link to obtain hotel accommodations. As a volunteer, I would not have to pay for the expenses, she explained.

This is happening really quickly. I wondered if I would still have to pay up front for the airline reservation. She asked me if I had any other considerations or concerns.

"Yes. I have a willing and able nineteen-year-old daughter, Caroline, who wants to come volunteer too. Is that possible?"

"Yes! She's an adult, and we would be happy to have her."

She hung up, and I began making plans. True to her word, the airline was very accommodating. All I needed to do was state that Caroline and I were volunteering in New York City, and the airline representative believed me. Our tickets and baggage would be paid for. About forty-five minutes later, I received an email confirming our reservation for La Quinta Inn in Central Park.

We both needed to pack. Since I had been traveling for work the past three years, I already had two suitcases for myself, but Caroline needed to purchase another. I worked that night at the hospital, but I obtained coverage and got off early.

I set the alarm for 5:00 a.m., but I was awake until 2:00 a.m. searching the internet for anything I could read about what was known so far about treating COVID-19 patients. There wasn't much to discover. I found some anecdotal stories I could read, but the literature was sparse. I just had to have faith that I would learn from the other doctors and acclimate quickly.

On the drive to Tulsa International Airport, Caroline and I finally had time to talk. Like me, Caroline loves New York City and everything about it; at one time she was even trying to launch her modeling career there. She was aware of how bad things were there now and was mindful that the city was overwhelmed. Granted, she wanted to further her career in New York City and check out the Fashion Institute of Technology, but she also wanted to help in any way she could at the hospital.

She asked me what I thought they would have her do. I told her they would probably just put her to work wherever they needed a helping hand. Even though of course she wished we were going there for fun, I could see how important it was to her that she was coming with me to help victims of the pandemic.

At the airport, I introduced myself at the United Airlines desk as Dr. Guinnip; destination: New York City, LaGuardia Airport. The attendant asked if I was going as a frontline worker, and I said yes.

"It takes special people like you two to leave home and go help others," she said.

Tears welled up in my eyes. Up until that point, it hadn't hit me that this was really happening. I had sat on my couch for about three weeks waiting for that anticipated phone call. Now it was happening. I hoped I could withstand this emotion. I realized how scared I was. *What if I get the virus? What if Caroline gets it?* But I really didn't think that fear would stop me now. Regardless, this was bigger than the two of us. No one in our family had been anything but supportive. *Now the time has come. This is why I became a doctor.*

I hoped that Caroline would not succumb to the virus. I had instructed her on how to use the personal protective equipment (PPE), and I constantly stressed wearing a mask, using hand sanitizer, washing her hands for at least twenty seconds, and keeping a distance of at least six feet from anyone she contacted. She complied well.

Nothing was open in the airport except one coffee shop; it was still early, and there were few travelers anyway because of the pandemic. We got our coffee and went to the gate, where four other passengers were waiting, sitting far apart. We boarded smoothly, and no one said a word about our destination. I had thought someone might comment. The plane had a total of nine passengers, and we were all spread out. The flight was uneventful. Our landing in Houston was impressive in that I counted sixty-four grounded planes. That airport is usually so busy, but not that day, and we passed few people on our way to our next gate. As we waited, the gate attendant made an announcement on the loudspeaker. It was *really* loud.

"We have with us traveling today a frontline worker named Dr. Guinnip," he announced. He did not mention Caroline. "Thank you for your service," he said.

I looked up, and everyone was clapping for me. It made me very emotional, and I could not soak it in. *I haven't saved anyone's life yet. Why are you clapping for me?*

There were nineteen passengers en route to LaGuardia. It's a three-and-a-half-hour flight, so I took the time to read medical clips and blogs and took a nap. We arrived around 4:00 p.m. (EDT), and it felt like we were the only ones in the airport.

I had decided we would take a taxi rather than the subway, and I was glad we did. The taxi driver was a very nice man, about my husband, Carlisle's age. He quickly sized me up and must have determined I was a doctor, because he started listing all his risk factors for the disease. He told me he was obese, had diabetes, and had chronic obstructive pulmonary disease. His father, who lived in a nursing home, had not yet tested positive for the coronavirus, but the driver was really worried for him.

He told us this was the first ride for him all day and that he was really hurting to make a living. He would have talked past arriving at the hotel if I had let him. He was a typical New Yorker and made us feel right at home.

Caroline found a sandwich shop that was open for delivery, and we had salads delivered to our hotel. That was the only way to get food now.

We acquiesced to our tiny but paid-for room, and by then it was time for us to go to sleep. I was worried about the next day on so many accounts. I was worried we would not arrive on time or that we would not find the hospital. Constantly replaying in my mind was the daily news coverage of Governor Cuomo asking for ventilators and imploring people to come help. I was worried there would not be enough ventilators, nor enough PPE.

Despite all of this, thankfully I still got some rest.

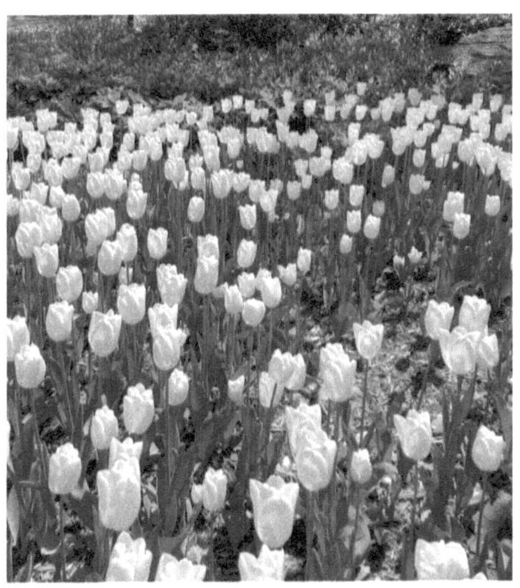

5

THE NEXT MORNING WAS A Monday, our first day as volunteers at North Central Bronx Hospital. Our subway ride went smoothly, though we still had to walk another mile to the hospital. When we arrived, a coordinator at the entrance asked us our post and shuffled us up to the eighth-floor command center. The command center was specifically set up for coronavirus patients and issues. There we obtained our badges and got some coffee.

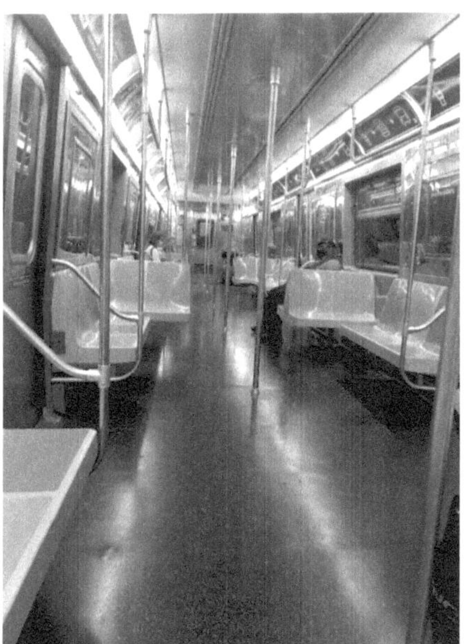

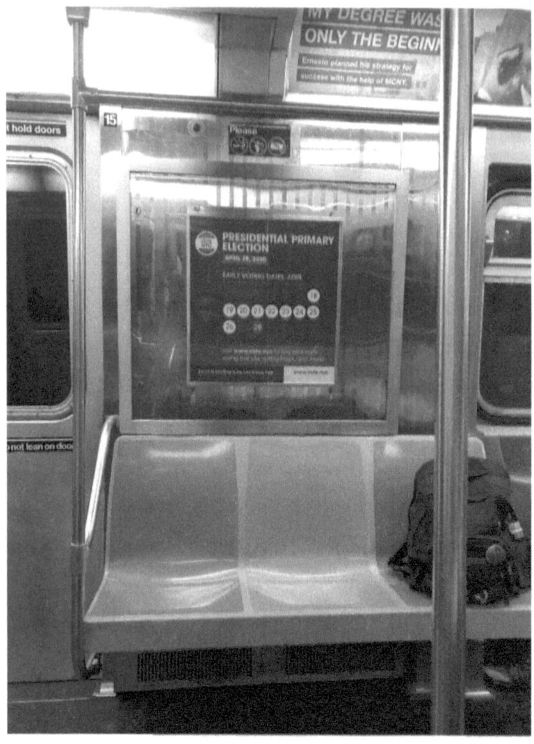

Robert, the gentleman who ran the command center, took to Caroline right from the start. He was so happy to have help and knew exactly what she could do each day. He directed her down to the lobby, where she would be posted that morning to provide nourishment to the staff. Chi-Chi soon walked in, greeted me warmly, and told me to head to the fourth floor, where there was a makeshift COVID-19 unit in the postanesthesia care unit (PACU).

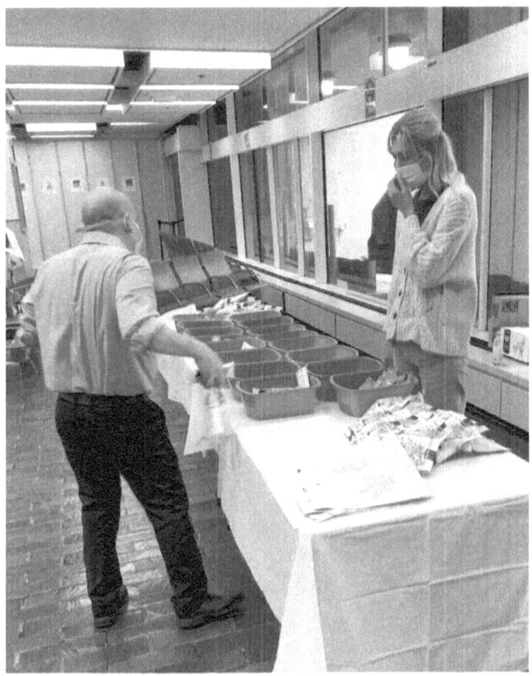

Outside the entrance to the unit were stacked boxes of PPE. I put my belongings in a locker, then put on the gear. Inside the unit I met Dr. Dimitrez, who up until then had been the chief of the unit. As a nephrologist, he was being transferred to another location where he could help with the surge of renal patients. He pointed me in the direction of the doctor who would give me sign-out, the important transfer of patient information. A semiretired pulmonologist, Dr. Pat Webster was volunteering as well. She walked me around the makeshift intensive care unit (ICU), giving me a rundown on the patients.

The first patient, a man in his sixties, was on a ventilator and on many medication drips. He was sedated heavily and looked very sweaty. The doctor told me she had been seeing a "stiff-lung" syndrome—likened to adult respiratory distress syndrome (ARDS)—which was requiring high oxygen levels and high pressure controls. This particular patient, previously healthy, had been transferred in from Coney Island and had been sick and on a ventilator since the middle of March. She listed all his medications, then asked me if I had any questions. At that point, I really didn't know what to ask. This was just the first patient.

The next patient was also around sixty, had been sick with COVID-19 since mid-March, and was also on a ventilator, requiring sedation and multiple drips. His settings were not that high, though, and Dr. Webster felt he was getting better. The third patient was not on a ventilator; around his late forties, he had been sick since mid-March and was getting a form of dialysis called CRRT (continuous renal replacement therapy). He was talkative and answered questions eagerly, and that was great to see.

I quickly learned that none of the New York City hospitals were allowing visitors; family members could only communicate via video chat calls, which they had to schedule a day in advance. This was true for patients with all types of illnesses, not just COVID-19. A nurse would bring the patient an iPad encased in a baggie to protect it, and the call would begin. Some of Caroline's eventual duties would include setting up these video chats, and I witnessed a few taking place during my time at the hospital.

There were five more patients in the unit, and Dr. Webster continued the rundown of their history. After she had finished, I received a call from Chi-Chi summoning me back to the command center. I was concerned, but at the command center, Chi-Chi just told me to finish my rounds with the pulmonologist and then go home, because she needed me back that night. She was switching me to the "Purple Zone," and I would be covering the night shift. That was not the best news, but *I guess I'll just have to deal with it.*

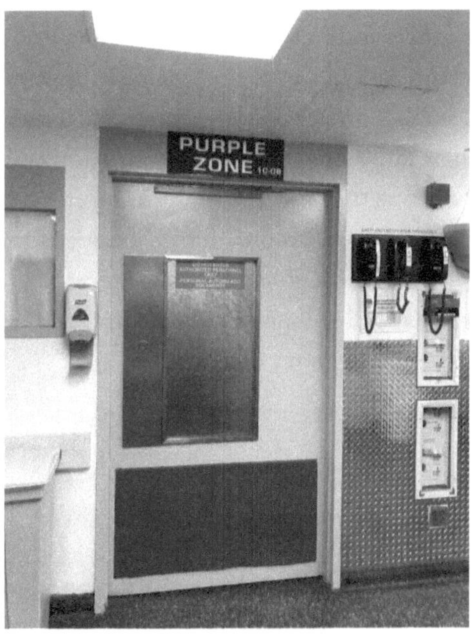

I texted Caroline and found out she had already gone back to our hotel in Manhattan via Uber, using some vouchers Robert had given her. She told me they were going to give me some vouchers as well. I was happy to hear that: taking the subway would have been a long trip to make each day. When I got back to the hotel, I learned that Caroline had spent her free time walking around Central Park, taking pictures, enjoying the sights, and going to the small grocery stores that were open. She seemed like she was having a great time. After I did some work on the computer, we spent the rest of the afternoon together.

Having Caroline there with me would turn out to be more helpful and enjoyable than I could ever have imagined. Besides working as a hospital volunteer, she would also act as my personal assistant. As the days passed, she made sure I had my morning coffee, and I could always look forward to a nice, healthy keto salad. Hospital staff members gave me a lot of positive feedback on her as well, saying what a go-getter she was and how impressed they were with her work ethic.

That day was the only day we spent together, but it was memorable. We walked around the desolate city and took pictures, saw the sights, and had fun being together. Of all the days I would spend volunteering, this day was the best day because I could be with my daughter.

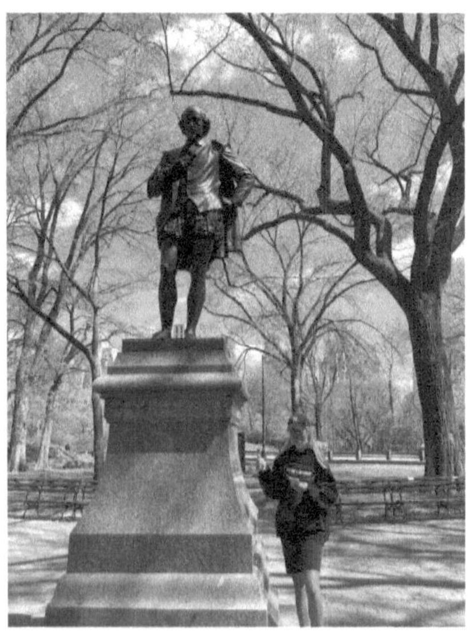

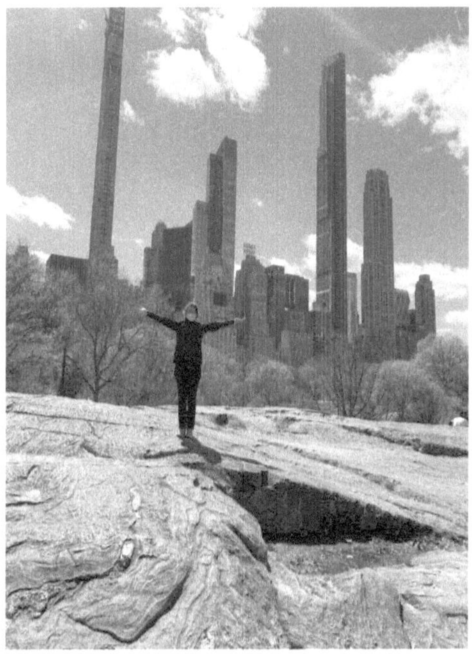

Later, I went back to the hotel to take a nap and prepare for the night shift.

6

THAT NIGHT I TOOK AN Uber back to the hospital. My shift started at 8:00 p.m., and I was assigned to the Purple Zone: a makeshift unit that was functioning as a COVID-19 emergency room.

After donning the PPE, I made eye contact with a doctor who needed to give me sign-out, and I had to exit the unit in order to do so. She introduced herself to me and said she was from Colorado. We got to know each other briefly, but I could sense she was worried because some patients were doing poorly. They were on the highest oxygen settings and still unstable. She quickly began transferring the patient information, signing out nine patients to me. As I had only been in the PACU for half the day, I did not have a lot of experience with COVID-19 patients. However, as the sign-out continued, the similarities among all the patients' stories became clear. These nine were all on ventilators, had contracted the coronavirus back in March, were heavily sedated, and were on multiple medications. They also all had stiff lungs consistent with ARDS.

Over the past weeks, this doctor had put together an algorithm to help manage the ARDS component. As she described it to me, it sounded extremely helpful; but unfortunately, few patients were getting better. It required oxygen at the maximum setting, and she was worried the patients might not recover.

As she continued her report, she told me that the unit had just started getting official consent from family members for patients to receive convalescent plasma transfusion (CPT) therapy. Only a few had received this new treatment thus far.

Before we made it too far into the sign-out, the nurse called us back in emergently: a patient was crashing. This patient was forty-two years old, had been transferred from Coney Island, and had severe ARDS, which required multiple intravenous inotropes (blood-pressure-elevating medication) and heavy sedation. Now he was bradycardic with a heart rate of 40, dropping quickly. He flatlined, and we started CPR. We ran the advanced cardiac life support protocol for thirty minutes until we were finally able to resuscitate him. My very first experience walking into the Purple Zone was a coding COVID-19 patient.

About an hour later, we finished sign-out, and she went back to her hotel to gear up for the morning. I went around to each patient and got to know them, got to know the nurse, drew labs, and made rounds every four hours. I only left to go to the bathroom. I met the other providers, including Christina (whom I quickly adopted as my nurse practitioner) and Odie, a trained CRNA (certified registered nurse anesthetist) currently functioning as a

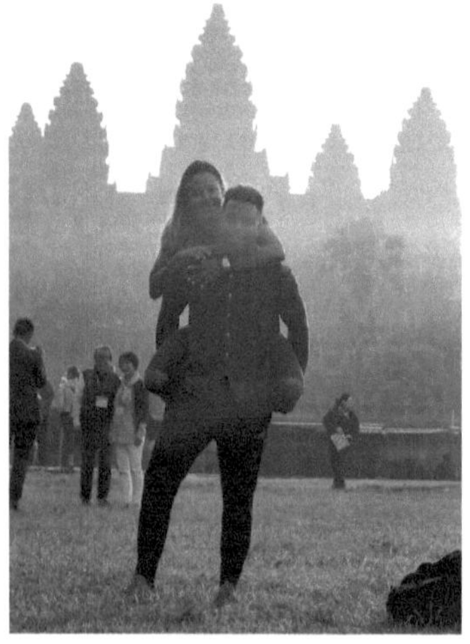

nurse practitioner. I met Dr. Harris (an anesthesiologist) and Nathalia (his significant other and nurse practitioner). Chi-Chi had arranged for some continuity in the schedule that week, so that we would be working with the same people and taking care of the same patients. The other nurses I came to know and work with were Jackie, Gabrielle, Hilda, and Pat. They were caring, empathetic, and smart.

The patient who had coded earlier had stabilized, but I had no idea if he would code again. I was on pins and needles throughout the night as I continued my rounds.

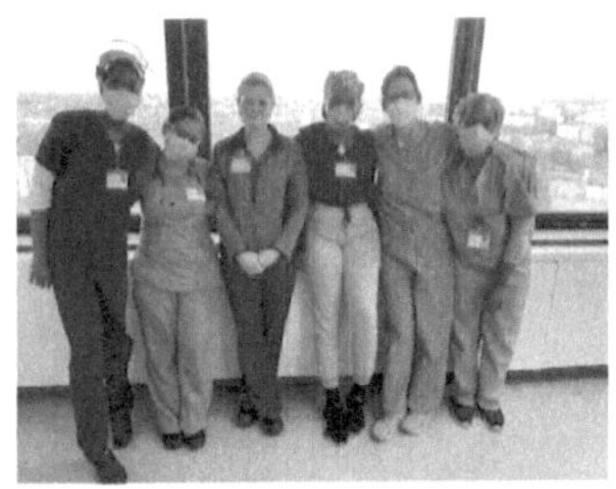

7

THE INITIAL SHOCK FOR ME was how sick these patients were. If I were to rate the illness's complexity and acuteness on a scale of 1 to 10, these patients were experiencing it at a 12. The growing number of cases also caused stress, but at least the influx of volunteers had reduced the number of patients per provider. I didn't get to know many local workers, because I spent all my time with fellow volunteers who had flown in from all over the United States—including Las Vegas, Nevada; Los Angeles, California; and Orlando, Tampa, and Jupiter, Florida. Our group was especially good about keeping up to date with the news and with all the scientific letters and papers that were coming out.

As the virus exponentially continued to infect people around the globe, doctors and scientists were collaborating and compiling data; they examined trends and common conditions seen to be associated with COVID-19, and they discussed possible treatment options. Because of the vast amount of cooperation among physicians and scientists, preliminary articles were being released from all around the world. Clinicians were quickly changing and updating their practices of treating these patients.

Miscommunication and extreme controversy arose about the safety and efficacy of hydroxychloroquine and azithromycin, the seeming promise of which had generated excitement both in the media and in the medical community. Four months into this disease, some anecdotal reports did seem to show improvement for patients who were early on in the disease. We also knew that chloroquine and hydroxychloroquine had been used in China and South Korea, reportedly with favorable results, although details were lacking. The initial promise of these drugs led to an emergency use authorization by the US Food and Drug Administration (FDA).

However, subsequent studies failed to show a significant benefit and highlighted the risk of QT prolongation, a syndrome that can lead to dangerous cardiac arrhythmias. As a result, the FDA revoked its emergency use authorization in mid-June, although some clinical trials are still in progress.[1] NIH guidelines recommend against the use of chloroquine or hydroxychloroquine in COVID-19 treatments except in the setting of a clinical trial; the NIH also cautions against the addition of azithromycin to hydroxychloroquine.[2] The WHO has a similar recommendation, and the Surviving Sepsis Campaign guidelines state that the data are insufficient to make a recommendation on the use of these agents.[3]

Another drug that has been getting some attention lately is remdesivir. I did not personally start this drug on any of my patients, but I know that some of them had been treated with it already. Remdesivir is an experimental antiviral agent with significant in vitro activity against coronaviruses[4] and some evidence of efficacy in an animal model of MERS-CoV (the Middle East respiratory syndrome-related coronavirus).[5] On May 1, the FDA issued an emergency use authorization for use of intravenous remdesivir to treat hospitalized patients with severe COVID-19, defined as having an oxygen saturation

(SpO2) of ninety-four percent or less on room air, requiring supplemental oxygen, mechanical ventilation, or extracorporeal membrane oxygenation (ECMO).[6] The WHO does not recommend its use outside clinical trials.[7]

In wide use during my time volunteering was CPT therapy. CPT stands for convalescent plasma therapy also known as neutralizing antibody. Every patient I treated either had received it already or received it after I obtained consent from their family. Studies on the therapeutic efficacy of CPT therapy are underway in various countries. In the United States, authorization must be obtained through the FDA.[8] The Infectious Diseases Society of America recommends CPT therapy for COVID-19 only in the context of a clinical trial.[9] Our work at the hospital was not yet part of a clinical trial, but the intention was that it would be.

Every patient was also being treated with dexamethasone, and I routinely placed patients on this drug. Preliminary data from a randomized clinical trial in more than six thousand hospitalized patients with COVID-19 found that dexamethasone reduced deaths in patients with severe respiratory complications requiring supplemental oxygen.[10] The details of the studied regimen have not been published, but the overall twenty-eight-day mortality rate was reduced seventeen percent in the dexamethasone group.[11]

As I mentioned, my very first experience attending to these patients was treating a patient presenting in cardiac arrest.

COVID-19 is a messenger-RNA virus. The virus brings the RNA (ribonucleic acid) into the cell, and the cell translates the RNA into a protein: in this case, a spike protein. This protein latches onto the ACE2 (angiotensin-converting enzyme 2) receptors that line various epithelial cell linings, including pulmonary, cardiovascular, and gastrointestinal tissues. One way the virus attacks the body is by binding to the cell receptors in these linings and destroying the cells it binds to. Interrupting this attaching mechanism has been one main way to target therapies thus far. A role for convalescent serum used in CPT is to provide antibodies that bind to the spike protein before it can attach to a cell and cause cell death.

The binding of the virus's spike protein to the cell receptor elicits a cascade of inflammatory chemicals as part of the body's natural immune response. This leads to a storm of inflammatory mediated cells (called a "cytokine storm") being released. Often, the resulting inflammation causes the release of even more of these inflammatory chemicals, resulting in a positive feedback cycle.

In the Spanish flu of 1918, the highest mortality rates were seen in the younger patients, in contradistinction to what we see with COVID-19. The inflammatory process in a young patient is robust; doctors and scientists theorize that in the Spanish flu, this immune response got amped up and continued in a never-ending positive feedback loop. In both pandemics, the common feature has been the elicitation of the cytokine storm, but we don't yet understand all the ways the inflammatory response to COVID-19 is causing multi-organ system failure.

Immune modulators such as dexamethasone can reduce the severity of the body's immune response by tempering the onslaught of the cytokine storm. This is T-cell-mediated and distinct from the antibody-mediated CPT. In addition to the dexamethasone treatment, other therapies have also been directed toward mitigating the cytokine storm and seem promising; however, more randomized trials are needed to show the benefits. Treatments that attack the virus specifically, called "antivirals," show promise as well.

One of the hallmarks we see with COVID-19 is ARDS, which often requires a patient to be placed on a mechanical ventilator.

The virus causes extreme damage to respiratory tissue. When the spike protein attaches to respiratory cells in the lungs, these cells die, and the body mounts a healing response, attempting to repair them. In this process, cells called macrophages and fibroblasts produce proteins (including collagen) to create scar tissue—tissue that can never revert to pulmonary tissue. That pulmonary tissue has been lost forever. So the patient's lungs become stiff, scar-like, and fibrotic. Once the patient is on a ventilator, the mortality rate is high: approximately eighty to ninety percent. This number likely reflects the fact that the scar tissue is not specialized to allow for oxygenation or ventilation.

Plain-film chest X-rays and CT scans of the chest have shown a common picture of diffuse reticulonodular infiltrates in both lungs, often in the bases and posterior. I was told by the doctors in New York that before coronavirus testing was widely available, as well as before test results were returned, doctors used the findings on these imaging modalities as a decision point regarding treatment. However, the American College of Radiology cautions that the findings on chest X-rays and CT chest scans are not specific to the novel coronavirus and overlap with other viral pneumonias.[12]

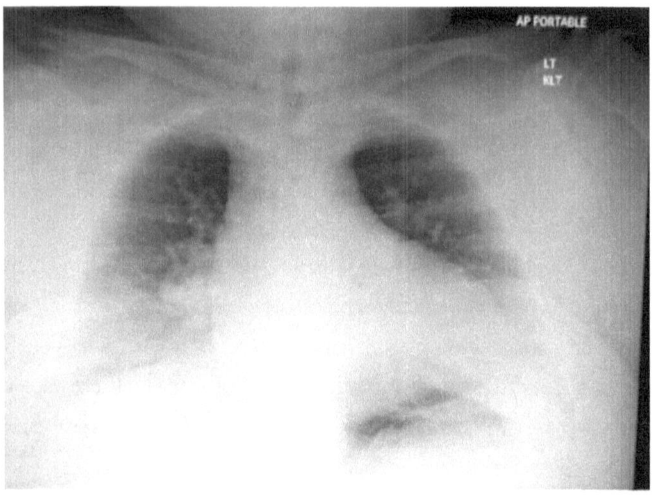

I quickly learned that managing a COVID-19 patient on a ventilator had unique challenges. Because the heart and lungs are one block and so interconnected, changing the settings on the ventilator to maximize oxygenation in the lungs can inadvertently decrease the heart's function. Making sure ventilator settings were optimal for each individual's needs was exhausting for the nurses, respiratory therapist, and physicians, and it necessitated frequent rounds. The previous doctors had thought that having the entire team round every four hours was a good place to start; however, some nights it was necessary to round on patients every hour.

Like the previous doctor, I was following the ARDSnet protocol for ventilator settings, but we ran into situations where there were no more settings we could turn to and nothing more we could do to help the patients' oxygenation. An idea brought up in March was to reposition the patients onto their stomachs (called "proning"), and it soon became part of the armamentarium. Guidelines and criteria (as well as a number to call to request the prone team) were posted on the wall. The method was to be used for patients who had been intubated for less than a week and had a PaO2/FiO2 ratio < 150 and FiO2 > 60%, PEEP > 10, as well as for any patient who their provider felt might benefit.

I treated ventilated prone patients, and the new method did help. The proning was likely allowing aeration of the back of the lungs and the bottom of the lungs—areas that previously were not being ventilated well. The proning enabled improved ventilation and aeration, but the patients' faces showed the damage from the pressure points. Once we started seeing the face wounds, we could implement preventative measures to unload those areas. The damage sustained during short amounts of time in the prone position contributed to the complications of necrosis.

The inflammatory cells released by the immune system can attack the heart muscle as well, causing the heart's electrical system and biological circuit to malfunction, resulting in ineffective pumping of blood. The inflammation also affects the arteries and veins that transport the blood, oxygen, and nutrients throughout the body. In a condition called endothelialitis, the damaged blood vessels become leaky, thus decreasing the volume of blood circulating throughout the body.

The blood pressure gets too low, and the organs essentially suffocate. COVID-19 patients have been seen to develop both the decreased heart function and the leaky vasculature that can ultimately lead to cardiovascular collapse and death, if not acted upon promptly. Because of the damage to the inner lining of blood vessels, clotting complications have been seen as well. Reports about treating these patients with blood thinners to mitigate the risks of clotting—although encouraging—are only anecdotal at this point.

I remember one patient who had very weak heart-muscle function when my shift began. By the end of the shift, though, he had improved and was even able to be weaned off some of his vasopressors. These medicines (which include norepinephrine, epinephrine, and dobutamine) support and increase blood pressure, and we were using them to treat him and the other patients requiring blood pressure support.

Physicians and scientists are actively working on antivirals that are showing some promise and that could potentially decrease the long-term cardiovascular complications that may arise from COVID-19, such as cardiomyopathy, arrhythmias, and coronary stenosis. To date (August 25, 2020), there are no specific studies to cite.

The coronavirus affects the renal system in a similar way, but the process has not yet been completely worked out. Doctors and scientists have hypothesized that the renal failure tends to occur concomitantly with the cardiovascular collapse, which in turn can be seen occurring hand in hand with severe respiratory failure (or shortly thereafter). The New York doctors informed me that they had been seeing a lot of renal failure in patients who were mechanically ventilated. These were anecdotal reports. Of the nine patients in the unit on my first night in the Purple Zone, those patients who had acute kidney injury had developed it concomitantly with their cardiovascular collapse. It is challenging enough for patients to suffer from COVID-19 while being mechanically ventilated with inotropes; undergoing renal replacement therapy, including dialysis, makes it all the more difficult. But there was no giving up.

Seeing all these complications made us aware that there was a fine line between giving a patient too much fluid (and overloading their heart), causing the fluid to back up and collect in the lungs and giving too little fluid. Over the course of my first week there, we honed in on a protocol for fluid management. Since COVID-19 was manifesting as ARDS, we avoided overhydration, feeling it would make the severe respiratory distress worse. Using transthoracic echocardiogram, which we had available at the bedside, we measured the change in cardiac output in response to fluid administration. One of the doctors taught me that you can assess fluid responsiveness by passive leg raising. An increase in cardiac output after one minute of passive leg raising has been shown to be a reliable predictor of response and helps to avoid overhydration in patients unlikely to respond.

Other patients I treated did not behave like they were critically ill. I gained some perspective on this after my first week. These patients looked well clinically, often occupying themselves doing crossword puzzles with no distress. However, their oxygen parameters were in a zone that made me very uncomfortable. Let me recall a sixty-two-year-old female with COVID-19. She had received CPT therapy and dexamethasone, and she was on twelve liters of nasal cannula oxygen. She was comfortable and not tachypneic (breathing abnormally rapidly), nor were her vital signs unstable; but her saturations were extremely low by traditional ICU standards (below 80%), and her arterial blood gas (ABG) showed a very acidotic pH (7.1) and arterial hypoxemia (54 mm of oxygen), as well as a bicarb of 22 with a high CO2. This ABG persisted for four days, then on the fifth day improved to a pH of 7.2. She got better, and we were able to wean her from her supplemental oxygen.

On the other hand, it was not uncommon to see the same ABG picture with a tachypneic patient who required mechanical ventilation. Why some patients worsened and deteriorated, sometimes within hours, and others stabilized is unknown. I hope the collaborating physicians researching this illness will get some answers eventually. The curious differences made taking care of these patients exceptionally difficult, especially since we didn't have any previous patient experience to go on. A navy physician who had treated patients in the PACU the week before my arrival told me he had a patient—previously stable—who had deteriorated suddenly and crashed. In many cases, the results were dismal.

Describing these patients makes me want to point out that COVID-19 does not usually progress to these situations. The illness ranges in severity from asymptomatic or mild to severe. Only about five percent of diagnosed cases require critical care to manage severe manifestations and complications, including ARDS, myocardial dysfunction, and shock.[13,14]

Thus far I have focused on patients I treated, but I do want to mention a staff member who contracted the coronavirus by working on the front lines. I got to hear her story directly. Pat, a registered nurse in the unit, told me that she had developed a fever of 100.8°F while working a long shift on April 8. She was not feeling well, and her supervisor sent her home that evening. She came back to the hospital the next day to be tested and was sure she had it even before the test came back positive. Prior to this she had been feeling exhausted but had attributed it to the long work hours due to the great influx of COVID-19 patients to the ICU.

Fortunately, although her illness protracted for two months before she was able to return to work, it was a mild case, and she beat it successfully. She is in her fifties and didn't have any other diseases (comorbidities), and prior to becoming ill, she had taken measures to stay in good health. She kept well-hydrated, exercised in the mornings, and kept her body strong from the inside out, drinking smoothies with nutritious ingredients to strengthen her immune response. She made sure to get rest the moment she arrived home each day, and she distanced herself from her family within the house so that her husband and two daughters would not (and thankfully did not) get it.

I asked her the best piece of advice she would want to give others. She stated that self-care is very important: you have to invest in treating your body well. She believes this has helped her fight off this and other illnesses.

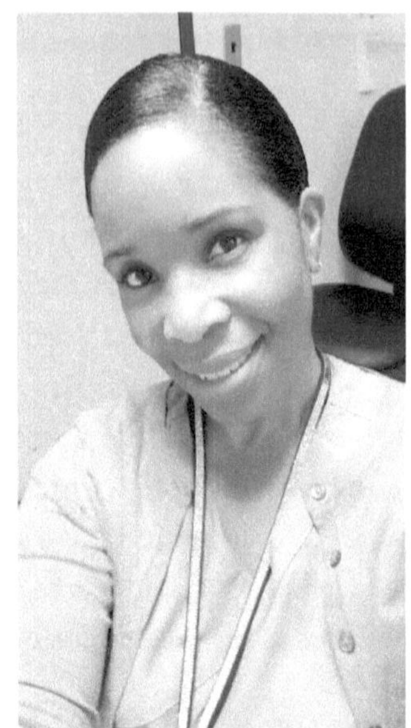 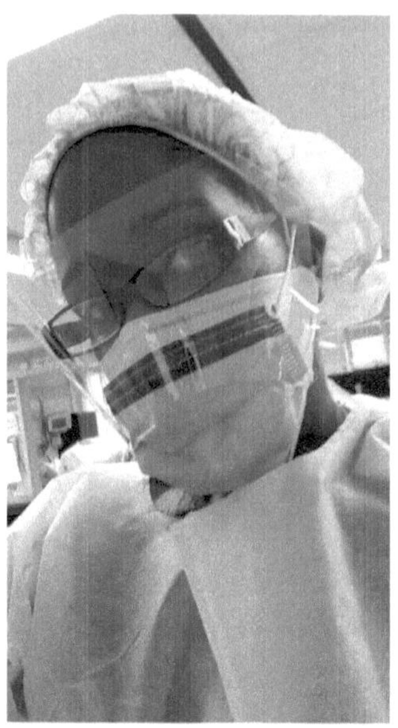

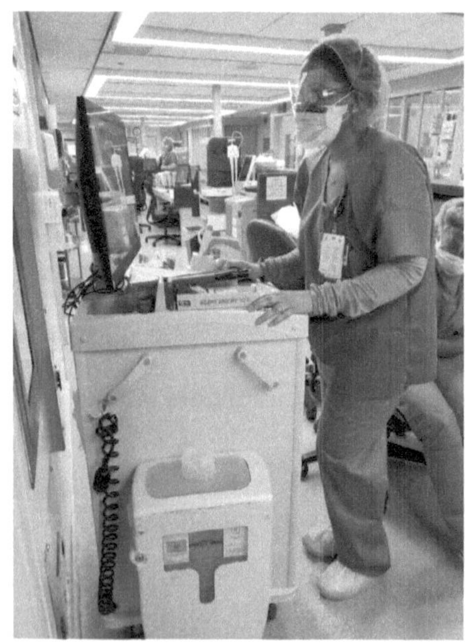

What struck me about Pat was her positive attitude. I would not have blamed her if she wanted to return to a different unit upon returning. As things stand, we are still not sure if a patient afflicted with COVID-19 is immune from becoming infected again. Regardless, Pat wanted to keep giving back. She was now uniquely qualified to empathize with her patients and their families. She made sure that patients and their families fully understood their care plan, and she encouraged their active involvement. I once saw her defuse a tense family disagreement with love, compassion, and patience. These humane, caring behaviors are often overlooked, nonprioritized, or even minimized in the face of strenuous circumstances. Pat has never forgotten the humanistic aspect of medicine. I have come to admire her, and I aspire to be like her.

8

THE ENTIRE GROUP OF NURSES and doctors that I worked with was composed of some of the most competent and thoughtful people I have ever encountered. Throughout our time together in the middle of a pandemic, we shared stories of how we were feeling and of how much we missed our families back at home. But our real worry was for New York and our ability to continue treating all its many patients suffering from COVID-19.

My fourth night in the Purple Zone, Chi-Chi sent her assistant, Tiana, to check on me. She donned her PPE and walked in around 11:45 p.m. with a message from Chi-Chi.

"Dr. G., are you able to continue to work here? Governor Cuomo has extended the disaster relief privileges until July 6. Do you think we can put you on the schedule in May? We could really use your help."

There was no sign of this slowing down. Nurses were being asked to stay longer. Christine, Odie, Nathalia, Dr. Harris, Jackie, and Gabrielle were all staying. They had become my team. It was only natural that I should stay too. Tiana told me I would be the doctor in charge with this same team again. We would keep working in the Purple Zone until construction was finished for our new coronavirus unit on the tenth floor, and another was being built on the fifteenth floor.

Maybe this is where I am supposed to be. Sure, it was a real "schlep" into work each day, as Chi-Chi referred to it, but I knew in my heart I had to make it. I was so excited. In the heat of the moment, I told Tiana I would be happy to come back.

I don't remember much of the rest of that night, but the next morning when I signed out to Dr. P., I felt so useful; I had a purpose. Dr. P. was a critical care physician volunteering from Los Angeles. I had met her my first night in the Purple Zone, and she was staying at La Quinta Inn as well. We had become friends instantly. After sign-out, I took an Uber back to the hotel, where Caroline had a mocha waiting for me. Then I went to sleep.

I was woken up by a phone call from Chi-Chi. She asked me how much I would want to work and told me I could stay on and work continuously. I asked her to allow me to go home first, but I promised I would come back as soon as possible. So she scheduled me for May. At this point I knew I needed to fly home with Caroline; the experience had overwhelmed me. But I was so happy to know I would be returning

This experience had been stressful, but it changed the moment I was asked to come back. It validated me and showed me that I was helping others and creating a positive environment for the team. Certainly, the hours were long, especially the night shift, but I started to settle in. Our team developed ways to cope with the circumstances. We developed goofy routines and made funny videos. It made each day of the seven-day assignment go by quickly.

An anticipated event was the walk to Tasty Picks. It was a dive to the locals, but it was our go-to to place for dinner during the night shift. The menu was vast, but what I liked the most was the chance to get out of the hospital for a break, to take the scenic walk two blocks to Gun Hill Road, and to breathe the New York air. I made it my priority to go often and would joyfully welcome one or two of the nurses to accompany me, most frequently Jackie and Gabrielle. We had time to goof off, tell jokes, and enjoy a small amount of down time.

The most memorable trek was the night it started snowing. It had been raining heavily, and we were all soaked through two layers of clothing. Suddenly, we felt snow crystals alight on our eyelashes. *This* was living. We changed our outer clothes when we got back and went back to the grind.

The next big event of the night was when I went around to the whole team and took their orders for Dunkin' Donuts. I usually made the donut run around 5:30 in the morning, so that I would have time to sign out with my team before I signed out to Dr. P. It amazed me how much joy a jelly donut could provide. The nurses loved the chocolate ones too. I loved going because I had fond memories of going as a young woman to the Dunkin' Donuts owned by my Uncle John in Auburn. It had been right next-door to my grandfather Beecher's home, and I had gone all the time to get snacks for my grandfather. He had been a widower for quite a while, and I had visited him as frequently as I could.

It touched my heart also because while I was volunteering, I got the sad news that Uncle John had passed away in a nursing home in Syracuse. He had been alone, with no one to hold his hand, when he took his final breath. The family was not even allowed to have a funeral because of the pandemic. I tried to be supportive to my aunt, but it was a challenging time. In the Purple Zone, I saw patients die without family members there to hold their hands, either. It felt so bizarre that family members couldn't visit. Video calls were their only means of communication with their loved one, and when the family started crying because their loved one did not respond or did not seem to recognize them, I would tear up underneath my three masks. Before I received news of my uncle's death, I had witnessed one of these heartbreaking video calls. I remember telling myself, *I can't imagine saying goodbye to a loved one that way.*

Then it happened to me. I did not find out until a few days after his death, and I felt torn and broken with no closure. I related to these family members of patients, understanding that they must have had the same feelings. Recalling my conversation with Pat just brought home to me the importance of relationships and the necessity of the support of family and friends. I watched our team providing necessary support to each other, and I watched the nurses do it multiple times every day. This became infectious and allowed us to get through each day.

As my time in April drew to a close, it was difficult to leave the patients and my team, but I took comfort in the fact that I was returning in a week. It had sunk in: I had done my part, and I would soon do more.

Caroline and I were flying home from Newark this time, and we had some crying spells on the taxi ride to the airport. We were both very sad to leave. I felt like I was abandoning the patients, even though it was not like that at all: Chi-Chi had found other doctors. But I felt like my heart would explode.

Our flight to Houston had about twenty passengers, but the flight to Tulsa had only about seven. When Caroline and I drove home, it felt like we had stepped into the twilight zone: the streets were full of vehicles, mainly trucks, in stark contrast to the bare city streets we had just left. Caroline pointed out how few people were wearing masks here, compared to nearly everyone in New York City. We would get a lot of scowls when we walked masked into Oklahoma convenience stores.

Upon arriving home, Caroline quarantined herself for two weeks. Restaurants had not yet opened, so she did not have to worry about going back to restaurant work yet.

I had tested negative for the coronavirus before leaving New York City, and I was feeling well. The governor of Oklahoma, Kevin Stitt, allowed frontline healthcare workers traveling from hot spots to go to work if they were well. By then, my local hospital wanted me back, asking me to work in the coronavirus unit because they could use the experience I had gained in New York City. I only worked a few days, however, before I was off to the Bronx for the second time.

My last night at home, I sat in my living room listening to the news, and once again I heard Governor Cuomo on a television commercial. These commercials were priceless, encompassing scenes of frontline workers doing their ordinary activities on the job. Governor Cuomo was thanking the nurses and doctors who were coming to New York City to help, and he stated that New York might be in the beginning of flattening the curve.

I went to play the piano, as I often did to gain perspective. Peace came over me like never before: I felt lucky; I felt like I mattered. I knew this trip back would be hard work, but I felt so relieved knowing there was a light at the end of the tunnel.

9

ON THE SECOND TRIP I went alone, and this time I stayed at a dicey hotel in the Bronx. I even think there were bullet holes in the wall!

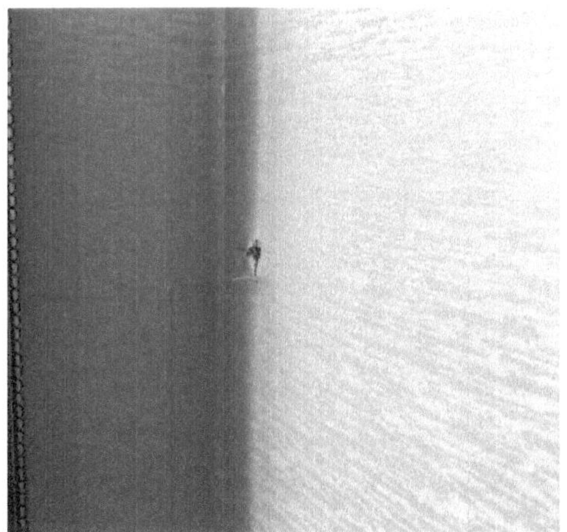

I took an Uber for every trip and quickly got into a routine. When I got back to my team Thursday night, big news was circulating: Hilda the nurse told me we were moving out of the Purple Zone to our new unit, 10A. We were so excited. During the day shift Thursday, the patients had all been moved upstairs.

Of our nine patients, one had died from complications of COVID-19, but the remaining eight were doing better. While I had been gone, general surgery had performed open tracheostomies on these patients to aid in weaning them off the ventilators. The patient who had coded on my first visit was still in critical condition but was being moved into the 10B ICU, a step-down unit. I was so happy to hear that. The other patients were still on ventilators, albeit with lower settings and out of the cytokine inflammation storm. Their vital signs were stable, and they required less vasopressor support. With their sedation being lifted, they were more interactive.

That Thursday night we all christened the new unit. It was an amazing improvement. The patients all had individual rooms, although, still, no visitors were allowed. PPE was stocked outside each patient's room, and the nurses and doctors had a very nice workstation. The best part is that we would not have to wear the N95 masks for twelve straight hours.

We transferred our exact routine from the Purple Zone, but now I was signing out to navy doctors from the USNS *Comfort*. Dr. P. had gone back to LA, but she called me daily to check on the patients. We still keep in touch now. The navy doctors were excellent, arrived early, and were an extreme joy to work with.

While we were signing out one day, the navy doctors told me that the USNS *Comfort* was leaving New York for good. We started to get the sense that the curve really was flattening in New York City. It was great! Even though the death rate took a few weeks to reflect the change, what we were doing—what we had put in place with our protocols—was working!

My mother and I had been enjoying weekly phone conversations for many years. When she heard that new cases in New York City were declining, she said to me, "It must be because of Paula!" What can I say about proud mothers?

This may sound awful, but with the curve flattening, I worried that my time would be over in New York City, because they would not need me anymore. Well, things did not translate so quickly into that kind of finality.

During my second week back, there were fewer new cases coming in and less chaos. The optimism was palpable. I continued the routine and made dinner trips and Dunkin' Donuts trips, but I had more time during the night. We all did. We could sit at the computers, read, listen to podcasts, and watch the news. Many binged Netflix content. Well, I am guilty as charged. I was able to binge-watch two seasons of *Better Call Saul*. This really worked to break up the time for me.

Then on a Saturday, Chi-Chi called and asked me to see Dr. Jessica S., as well as Drs. N. and R., before I left. With the curve seemingly flattening, this seemed like a concerning change of plans. However, Chi-Chi explained that these three women ran the ICU in 10B and were also in charge of staffing the new unit on the fifteenth floor. Then she asked if I wanted to work there on contract for six months with the Physician Affiliate Group of New York. I was thrilled.

Before I left for my plane that day, I went by and introduced myself to Dr. S. She was young, vibrant, and very smart and explained she needed help in 10B. Of course I would help! Then Dr. R. asked me if I would also work upstairs on the fifteenth floor, which was becoming another step-down unit. Certainly! The doctors could feel my enthusiasm.

I was so excited on my flight home. There were more passengers this time, though it was not yet fifty percent full. Back in Oklahoma things were starting back up in the operating room. I had not heard from my job in Missouri, so I stayed in Oklahoma. As I waited to be scheduled for my new position, I performed surgery again, saw patients in the office, and offered telemedicine visits. I was trying to adapt to the new normal. Around the middle of May I received an email from Dr. S. letting me know that they were scheduling me to cover 10B for ten days in June. I was so excited.

I continued working shifts at my local hospital until then and had time to really make plans. Things were better. New York City was starting to look like the poster child for all good things: cases were decreasing, and people were pulling through. I would be treating new coronavirus patients, patients still on ventilators, and patients who had multiorgan damage, but this trip back was nothing like my two previous visits.

This time, upstairs on 10B, the average age of my patients was fifty; they were all Latino and all male. By June the hospital had gone away from video chat calls, and now one family member could visit at a time. Two hours each day were designated for short visits of thirty minutes or less. There was more foot traffic now in the hospital, and it was more difficult to keep track of family members who were supposed to be practicing social distancing, wearing their masks, washing their hands, and using hand sanitizers.

I had residents who were finishing their first year of training. This new generation of doctors gives me great hope for the future. Having them around to teach them and to learn from them was the best part of my third visit. I love them.

Again, I had concerns that they would not need me to come back, and in my heart I was sure they wouldn't. But they said they would need ongoing help on the fifteenth floor as those patients recovered. True to their word, they scheduled me for July 6–17

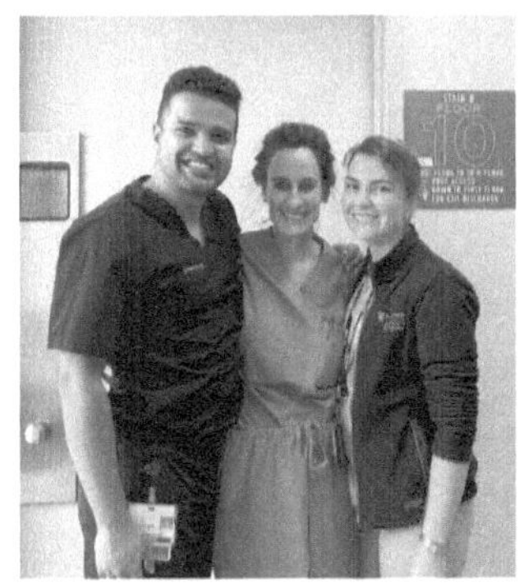

on the fifteenth floor. This floor was now an ICU filled with COVID-19 patients who were not yet ready to be discharged to a rehab unit or home. It was like a long-term acute-care facility within the hospital, and it would have been perfect for me, because I had worked in a long-term acute-care facility from 2017 through 2020. Then something happened that changed everything.

The cases in New York City had dropped so low that now Governor Cuomo had decided to restrict entry from thirteen states for fear of spreading the virus back to the recovering New Yorkers. Oklahoma was on that list. While this would not completely prevent me from returning, the policy required a two-week quarantine prior to going about business in New York. Unfortunately, I did not feel that was doable. My family will tell you I cried the whole day when I heard the news. I had my heart set on my new phase of life, treating COVID-19 patients in New York City, but now it was not happening.

I am still not happy about this, but suffice it to say that my trips to New York City were the best and most rewarding experiences I had ever had since become a physician twenty-eight years ago and a cardiac surgeon twenty years ago. It has changed me in a New York minute.

I have always admired Dr. Fauci. I was once jealous of my fellow classmate from Georgetown, Dr. Mark Dybul, who has worked for his whole career with Dr. Fauci and will probably become the "next Dr. Fauci." I am the biggest Yankee fan you will ever come across, and when Dr. Fauci was lucky enough to throw out the first pitch on the opening day of Major League Baseball's 2020 season—when the Yankees played the World Series 2019 Champion, the Nationals—I was green with envy. Shame on me for feeling that way.

Dr. Fauci has been stellar throughout this and all pandemics for the past fifty years, and when he threw out that first pitch, I was so happy for him. I am so proud of him and his accomplishments.

At 7:00 p.m. every night during those trying months, everyone in all of New York City would let out a "primal scream" in solidarity for all the workers fighting the pandemic. I remember participating in my own primal scream thirty-five years ago after finishing a grueling exam at Cornell. As luck would have it, I got a special moment when the Yankees (in a stadium without any fans) honored the frontline workers. At 7:00 p.m. on MLB's opening day, July 23, 2020, the Yankees let out their own primal scream, banging cans and lids with their bats and making noise to honor the doctors and nurses who had helped in the pandemic. Need I say more? There was no greater moment for me. One day soon, hopefully when they are playing in the World Series, I want to journey back to the Bronx to Yankee Stadium and thank the team and organization personally.

What Caroline and I were part of was bigger than we had ever dreamed. We were two people trying to do our best to help others. I thank God I had the courage to respond to the first email Governor Cuomo sent out. Had I not gone outside my comfort zone, I do not think I would have appreciated the magnitude of the effect that this pandemic has had on us all. I never thought I would be working, struggling, and sweating through a once-in-a-lifetime global crisis, in one of the most devastated places on earth, with some of the most courageous and honorable people I have ever known. That New York minute expanded my thinking, opened me up to new experiences, and renewed me as a human being and as a physician.

Acknowledgments

I HAVE TO THANK FROM the bottom of my heart the great doctors, nurses, and staff members with whom I worked: Dr. Joy, Dr. Pandhiri, Dr. Lacey, Dr. Harris, Dr. Steven, Dr. Christian, Dr. Kevin, Dr. Anyaogu, Dr. Stoeckel, Dr. Dominique, Dr. Ramasamy, Dr. Nalamati, Dr. Pradhan, Jackie, Gabrielle, Hilda, Pat, the internal medicine residents of the North Central Bronx Hospital, the radiology technologists, the unit managers, the ER managers, and the command center staff. Thanks also to all the friendly Lyft and Uber drivers I met along the way.

I also want to thank Alicia Keys for recording her song "Good Job" and Jon Bon Jovi for coming on the local radio station every night during the early months and saying thank you to the frontline workers. I want to mention the cast of *The Five* on Fox News and thank them for making me smile.

I also have to thank my family, including Carlisle and Gunnar for supporting me and allowing me to go to New York City. I missed Logan; my firstborn daughter, Elizabeth; and my grandson, Lake, so much. Having to see my grandson on FaceTime from the beginning of his life has been difficult. I do not want to subject any of them to the risk of COVID-19, so I don't know when I will see him again. I want to thank my parents and God for giving me life, and my grandparents for making me feel I could achieve anything as long as I did not weaken. All of these beloved family members helped raise me.

And most importantly, I want to thank you, the reader, for allowing me to share my story. I hope you enjoyed this small excerpt from my fifty-three years and the story of this experience, which has become the best and most purposeful time of my life.

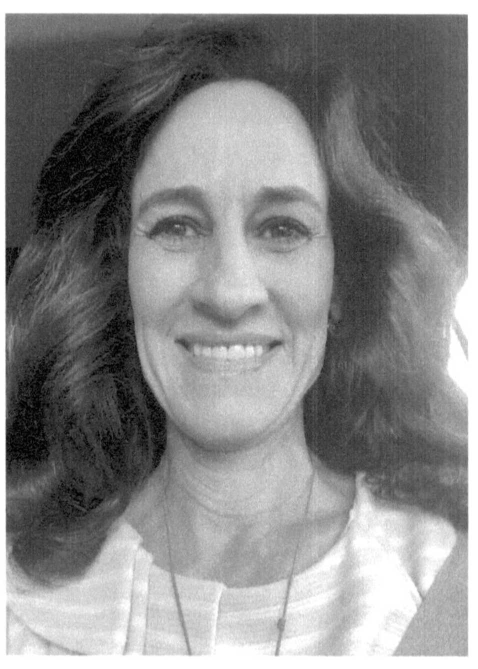

References

1. Gao, J., et al. "Breakthrough: Chloroquine Phosphate Has Shown Apparent Efficacy in Treatment of COVID-19 Associated Pneumonia in Clinical Studies." Letter to the editor. *Bioscience Trends* 14, no. 1 (2020): 72–73.

2. National Institutes of Health. "COVID-19 Treatment Guidelines." Updated June 25, 2020. Accessed June 29, 2020. NIH website.

3. World Health Organization. "Clinical Management of COVID-19: Interim Guidance." Updated May 27, 2020. Accessed June 29, 2020. WHO website.

4, 5, 6, 7. Food and Drug Administration. "Fact Sheet for Health Care Providers: Emergency Use Authorization (EUA) of Remdesivir (GS-5734)." Updated June 2020. Accessed June 29, 2020. FDA website.

8. Food and Drug Administration. "Recommendations for Investigational COVID-19 Convalescent Plasma." Updated May 1, 2020. Accessed June 29, 2020. FDA website.

9. Bhimraj, A., et al. "Infectious Disease Society of America Guidelines on the Treatment and Management of Patients with COVID-19." Published April 11, 2020. Updated June 25, 2020. Accessed June 29, 2020. IDSA website.

10, 11. Chief Investigators of the Randomized Evaluation of COVid-19 thERapY (RECOVERY) Trial on Dexamethasone. "Low-Cost Dexamethasone Reduces Death by up to One Third in Hospitalized Patients with Severe Respiratory Complications of COVID-19." Updated June 16, 2020. Accessed June 29, 2020. RECOVERY Trial website.

12. American College of Radiology. "ACR Recommendations for the Use of Chest Radiography and Computed Tomography (CT) for Suspected COVID-19 Infection." Updated March 22, 2020. Accessed June 29, 2020. ACR website.

13, 14. Centers for Disease Control. "Coronavirus Disease 2019 (COVID-19): Interim Clinical Guidance for Management of Patients with Confirmed Coronavirus Disease (COVID-19)." Updated May 29, 2020. Accessed June 29, 2020. CDC website.